PMPs for the MRCPsych Part II

by

Dr Michael I. Levi MB, BS, MRCPsych

with a Foreword by
Dr D G Walbridge
Consultant Psychiatrist, Royal South Hants Hospital,
Southampton, UK

KLUWER ACADEMIC PUBLISHERS
DORDRECHT / BOSTON / LONDON

Distributors

---

for the United States and Canada: Kluwer Academic Publishers, PO Box 358, Accord
Station, Hingham, MA 02018-0358, USA
for all other countries: Kluwer Academic Publishers Group, Distribution Center, PO Box
322, 3300 AH Dordrecht, The Netherlands

British Library Cataloguing in Publication Data is available

ISBN 0-7923-8993-X

Contents

Foreword   vii

Introduction   ix

Examination Technique   xi

Patient Management Problems 1–40   1

Foreword

Recent years have seen many changes in the format of the MRCPsych examinations and candidates are indeed fortunate to have the works of Dr Levi as a guide to what awaits them and as an aid to preparation. The dreaded multiple choice and short answer questions have already been addressed by the author and now comes the turn of the Patient Management Problems viva. In this, the aspiring psychiatrist will be presented with perhaps three or four clinical vignettes and invited to discuss their immediate thoughts on diagnosis and management. This seems to me to be a clear advance on the previous format of being interrogated, after the fashion of Mastermind, for thirty minutes on progressively obscure aspects of psychiatric knowledge and much more representative of what constitutes competence in clinical practice. No longer will it be sufficient preparation to swallow large textbooks with the intention of later regurgitating the relevant information in undigested form: a different emphasis in revision is obviously necessary.

Here then, is a guide to that revision: 40 specimen vignettes over a wide range of problems with suggested answers. The reader should study each problem, consider their answer, then turn the page and see how they fared. Of course, they will not always agree with Dr Levi's answer and, for example, might decide that the gentleman in Question 14 is more likely to be suffering from a further relapse of his schizophrenia than anything else or that their own preferred diagnosis in Question 40 would be one of depression with panic attacks. Agreement or not is immaterial, however, as in disagreeing one is forced to justify one's own line of thought in exactly the same way as the examiners will later demand, and if argument and thought can be thus provoked and practised then the likelihood of depression with panic attacks during the examination is considerably less. What no-one can disagree with is the necessity of adopting a multi-disciplinary approach to assessment and all of the answers show how this might be structured. See, for example, Question 31 for a paradigm of all-round management of an all-too-familiar scenario.

Just for good measure, the fine print has not been neglected and conditions such as de Clerambault's syndrome, dysmorphophobia and monosymptomatic delusional psychosis are described and discussed. Probably, few candidates will have seen all three in pure form and it is worth remembering that uncommon conditions occur rather more commonly during examinations than in the clinic or the casualty department, where the sound of hoofbeats, to borrow an American phrase, only rarely indicates the presence of a zebra. So the more it changes, the more it stays the same: you still have to read the large textbooks.

Enough of metaphors, especially American ones, and on to the examination technique. Dr Levi has included some helpful tips on addressing the Patient Management Problems and the wise candidate will do well to follow them. Having done so, gather together fellow examinees and request practice viva sessions with senior colleagues. There really is nothing like repeated practice for sharpening up presentation and, as an added bonus, it desensitizes anxiety in that, having been embarrassed and tormented in the presence of one's peers, the examination itself is an almost pleasurable experience. A cheerful and confident manner can only impress the examiners and with any luck they will have read this book as well to help them make up their questions.

D.G. Walbridge
Consultant Psychiatrist,
Royal South Hants Hospital,
Southampton, UK

Introduction

A major component of the MRCPsych Part II examination for Membership of the Royal College of Psychiatrists is the inclusion of a Patient Management Problem (PMP) oral examination. The candidate has to answer 4 or 5 questions in 30 minutes. The questions are on clinical topics in psychiatry.

The purpose of writing this book is to give candidates adequate practice at the types of PMP they will encounter. I have based these PMPs on what is generally regarded to be the most easily readable and evenly written textbook[1] for the MRCPsych examination. The 40 PMPs in this book cover the full range of psychiatric practice.

Reference

1. Gelder, M., Gath, D. and Mayou, R. (1989). *Oxford Textbook of Psychiatry*, 2nd Edition (Oxford: Oxford Medical Publications)

Examination Technique

1. Having been presented with the PMP by the examiners, start by saying how you would take a full history, perform a mental state examination and do a full physical examination, focussing on those areas relevant to making a diagnosis.

2. Continue by saying that you would obtain more information by speaking to informants or the patient's GP, by getting the old case notes and by obtaining reports from other agencies (e.g. employer).

3. Next state how you would wish to carry out further assessments in the form of physical investigations, a social worker's report, a family interview, psychometry, observations by nursing staff and occupational therapy assessments as appropriate to the case.

4. Continue by giving your preferred (i.e. most likely) diagnosis and differential diagnoses.

5. Finally, give your management of the diagnosis given.

In the answers to the PMPs in this book, I have assumed that the candidate will mention points one to three above at the beginning of their answer each time, before going on to aspects of differential diagnosis and management. The same principle applies to the actual examination. However, after answering the first PMP presented by the examiners in this way, it may be acceptable to answer the subsequent PMPs by immediately stating your preferred diagnosis, differential diagnosis and management of the diagnosis given in the interests of time.

Question 1

- 65-year-old man

- Referred from Casualty for a psychiatric opinion

- History of three previous psychiatric admissions in the last thirty years for depressive disorder

- Presents with a one-week history of believing his wife is plotting against him, believing he is the Messiah, sexual disinhibition and agitation

- Also presents with a two-day history of confusion and alcohol abuse

- What is the differential diagnosis and management of this patient?

Answer 1

(a) *Differential diagnosis –*

– Hypomania – most likely diagnosis

– Need to consider senile dementia and alcohol intoxication

(b) *Management –*

– Admit patient to hospital for further assessment

– Immediate management – major tranquilizers in carefully titrated doses

– If the patient subsequently develops clear-cut depressive symptoms – consider a non-cardiotoxic antidepressant drug, e.g. fluvoxamine (a 5-HT reuptake inhibitor)

– If the patient fails to respond to antidepressant medication – consider a course of ECT

– If the patient fails to respond to the above treatment – consider a trial of lithium carbonate, aiming for a serum lithium level of approximately 0.4 mmol/L for maintenance treatment

Question 2

- 22-year-old lady

- Referred from Casualty for a psychiatric opinion

- History of two previous psychiatric admissions for attempted suicide in the form of wrist slashing

- History of alcohol and drug abuse, sexual abuse by her step-father, and a forensic history for shoplifting

- Presents with a three-week history of feeling depressed, loss of energy, constipation, loss of appetite and feeling suicidal

- Shortly prior to attendance at Casualty, she attempted to overdose on paracetamol tablets but was stopped by her boyfriend

- What is the differential diagnosis and management of this patient?

Answer 2

(a) *Differential diagnosis* –

- Antisocial personality disorder – most likely diagnosis

- Need to consider depressive disorder

(b) *Management* –

- Admit to hospital for further assessment including assessment of suicidal risk

- Identify the psychosocial stresses in the patient's life and try to manipulate them where possible

- If patient fails to respond to pyschosocial manipulation, antidepressant medication may subsequently be indicated

- If patient motivated, consider:

    (i) Referral to a therapeutic community

    (ii) Ongoing supportive psychotherapy (either individual or group) aimed at helping the patient to recognize her problems and relate in a mature responsible manner to individuals and society

Question 3

-   70-year-old lady

-   Referred by her GP to the Outpatients' Department

-   No previous psychiatric admissions

-   Husband died five months ago

-   Presents with a three-month history of sadness, yearning for the deceased, preoccupation with thoughts of the deceased, loss of appetite, loss of weight and sleep disturbance

-   What is the differential diagnosis and management of this patient?

Answer 3

(a) *Differential diagnosis* –

–   Grief reaction – most likely diagnosis

–   Need to consider depressive disorder

(b) *Management* –

–   Admit to hospital for further assessment – including assessment of
    the degree of depression

–   Initiate bereavement counselling in hospital with one of the ward
    nurses trained in counselling skills

–   After discharge, bereavement counselling can be continued by a
    Community Psychiatric Nurse

–   If clinically depressed, treat with an antidepressant drug

–   If patient fails to respond to antidepressant medication, consider a
    course of ECT

–   Follow up in the Outpatients' Department and continue
    antidepressant medication for six months post-clinical recovery for
    prophylaxis

Question 4

- 50-year-old lady

- Referred by her GP to the Outpatients' Department

- No previous psychiatric admissions

- Presents with a one-year history dominated by repeatedly checking to ensure that gas and water taps are turned off, and that windows and doors are shut, becoming increasingly anxious if she doesn't carry out these checking rituals

- At times she also experiences feelings of depression and irritability

- What is the differential diagnosis and management of this patient?

Answer 4

(a) *Differential diagnosis* –

– Primary OCD (obsessive compulsive disorder) – most likely diagnosis

– Need to consider depressive disorder with marked secondary obsessive compulsive symptoms

(b) *Management* –

– Treat patient as an outpatient with a drug which specifically targets obsessional symptoms, e.g. fluvoxamine (a 5-HT reuptake inhibitor)

– To deal with compulsive rituals, a behavioural approach might be attempted with exposure and response prevention, i.e. by exposing the patient to those situations previously evoking checking behaviour and persuading her to refrain from carrying out the rituals – with persistence, the rituals and the distress may subsequently diminish

– Supportive psychotherapy may benefit the patient by providing continuing hope

– In planning treatment, it is essential to interview other family members and encourage them to adopt a firm but sympathetic attitude to the patient

Question 5

- 50-year-old man

- Referred by his GP to the Outpatients' Department

- History of three previous psychiatric admissions for detoxification from alcohol

- Presents with a one-month history of impairment of recent memory, confabulation and retrograde amnesia with no impairment of consciousness

- What is the differential diagnosis and management of this patient?

Answer 5

(a) *Differential diagnosis –*

- Korsakoff's psychosis associated with alcohol dependence – most likely diagnosis

- Need to consider pre-senile dementia due to other possible causes

(b) *Management –*

- Admit patient to hospital for further assessment

- The patient should have a full physical examination and full physical investigations to assess the extent of alcohol abuse

- Detoxify from alcohol with a chlormethiazole or chlordiazepoxide reducing regime

- Vigorous treatment with parenteral thiamine may produce some degree of recovery in his memory deficits

- Rehydrate if patient has any electrolyte imbalance

- Give glucose if patient has any hypoglycaemia

- Give antibiotics if patient has any infection

- Give anticonvulsants if patient has any convulsions, e.g. large doses of chlordiazepoxide

- Advise patient to totally abstain from alcohol and counsel him about the physical, social and psychological complications of alcohol dependence

- Attend to any accompanying problems the patient may have in his health, marriage, job or social adjustment

- Recommend the patient to try Alcoholics Anonymous

- Recommend the patient to try using a diary and other memory aids, which may produce some degree of compensation for the memory deficits

Question 6

- 49-year-old lady

- Referred by her GP for an urgent outpatient's appointment

- History of three previous psychiatric admissions over the last four years – diagnosed at different times as suffering from schizophrenia, schizoaffective disorder and hypomania, remaining fairly well in between admissions

- Presents with a one-month history of believing she is the most intelligent person in the world, hearing voices telling her that she has special powers, experiencing that others can 'read' her thoughts, and hearing a voice speaking her thoughts as she thinks them

- What is the differential diagnosis and management of this patient?

Answer 6

(a) *Differential diagnosis* –

– Schizoaffective disorder (schizomania) – most likely diagnosis

– Need to consider schizophrenia and hypomania

(b) *Management* –

– Admit to hospital for further assessment (including observations by nursing staff on the ward)

– Immediate management – chlorpromazine in moderate doses

– Long-term management – depot antipsychotic medication (e.g. haloperidol decanoate) and lithium carbonate required for prophylaxis

– Follow up patient frequently at the depot clinic

Question 7

-   36-year-old lady

-   Referred by her GP to the Outpatients' Department

-   History of two previous psychiatric admissions for anxiety neurosis and phobic anxiety neurosis respectively

-   Presents with a one-year history of worsening of agoraphobic symptoms culminating in the patient becoming housebound and extremely anxious

-   What is the differential diagnosis and management of this patient?

Answer 7

(a) *Differential diagnosis –*

– Primary phobic anxiety neurosis (agoraphobia) – most likely diagnosis

– Need to consider a primary anxiety neurosis with secondary phobic symtoms

(b) *Management –*

– Treat patient with a form of systematic desensitization, administered by a clinical psychologist

– Gradually encourage the patient to walk increasing distances from her house – in the company of the psychologist

– The patient should also be taught relaxation training and anxiety management training and encouraged to practice these at home

– It may be necessary to augment psychological treatment with:

   (i) Anxiolytic medication (e.g. short-term use of a benzodiazepine); or

   (ii) An MAOI (e.g. phenelzine); or

   (iii) The tricyclic antidepressant imipramine (which some clinicians consider to be the treatment of choice for agoraphobia)

Question 8

-   25-year-old lady

-   Referred from a maternity ward for a psychiatric opinion, having delivered her first child one week ago

-   No previous psychiatric admissions

-   Presents with an acute onset of believing her family are against her, depressed mood, muddled and illogical conversation, ideas of hopelessness and inappropriate laughter

-   What is the differential diagnosis and management of this patient?

Answer 8

(a) *Differential diagnosis –*

– Puerperal psychosis (schizoaffective type) – most likely diagnosis

– Need to consider puerperal psychosis (schizophrenic or affective type)

(b) *Management –*

– Transfer patient to a psychiatric unit with facilities for admission of the baby (i.e. a mother-and-baby unit) to enable 'bonding'

– Allow the patient to maintain contact with her baby and to care for it, under supervision

– Breast feeding may be continued where possible

– Treatment of the psychosis inside the puerperium is the same as that for psychosis occurring outside the puerperium

– Since this patient presents with a schizoaffective type of puerperal psychosis, treatment with a neuroleptic and an antidepressant would be appropriate

– If the response to antidepressant medication is slow, a course of ECT should be considered

– Following improvement, the patient should be allowed on increasing amounts of leave with her baby, with a view to early discharge

– Follow up in the Outpatients' Department

Question 9

- 75-year-old socially isolated man

- Referred by his GP to the Outpatients' Department

- No previous psychiatric admissions

- Presents with a one-month history of loss of appetite, loss of weight, poor attention and concentration, memory impairment and agitation

- What is the differential diagnosis and management of this patient?

Answer 9

(a) *Differential diagnosis* –

– Depressive disorder with pseudodementia – most likely diagnosis

– Need to consider senile dementia

(b) *Management* –

– Admit to hospital for further assessment

– Treat patient with a sedative antidepressant drug, e.g. Prothiaden

– If patient fails to respond to antidepressant medication, consider a course of ECT

– Encourage patient to attend the psychogeriatric day hospital following discharge, to:

    (i)   Reduce his social isolation

    (ii) Allow his mental state to be monitored

    (iii) Check on his compliance with medication

Question 10

– 35-year-old lady

– Taken to Casualty on Section 136 of the Mental Health Act
   (MHA) 1983 by the police – found exposing herself in public

– History of three previous psychiatric admissions over the last seven
   years – diagnosed at different times as suffering from
   schizophrenia, depressive disorder and schizoaffective disorder;
   remaining well in between admissions

– Presents with overactivity, elated mood, rapid and copious speech,
   rapidly changing topics of conversation and lack of insight

– What is the differential diagnosis and management of this patient?

Answer 10

(a) *Differential diagnosis* –

- Hypomania – most likely diagnosis

- Need to consider schizophrenia and schizoaffective disorder

(b) *Management* –

- In view of the acutely disturbed behaviour – admit to hospital

- May need to detain under the MHA 1983

- Immediate management – haloperidol (oral or parenteral) in moderate to large doses

- Long-term management – lithium carbonate required as a mood stabilizer for prophylaxis

- Follow up patient frequently at the Outpatients' Department

Question 11

- 26-year-old lady

- Referred from Casualty for a psychiatric opinion

- No previous psychiatric admissions

- Presents with a three-week history of believing that the film star Richard Gere, with whom she has had no contact, is in love with her and made the initial advances; for the last week she has been trying to phone him in Los Angeles, California; this belief does not appear to be associated with any other disorder

- What is the differential diagnosis and management of this patient?

Answer 11

(a) *Differential diagnosis* –

- De Clerambault's syndrome ('pure' form) – most likely diagnosis

- Need to consider schizophrenia, affective disorder and organic disorder

(b) *Management* –

- Admit to hospital for further assessment

- If underlying disorder present – treat it appropriately

- If 'pure' form – very resistant to physical treatment and psychotherapy

- Follow up in the Outpatients' Department

Question 12

- 25-year-old lady

- Taken to Casualty on Section 136 of the Mental Health Act 1983 by the police – found trying to jump onto the rails in a tube station, having to be restrained by members of the public

- No previous psychiatric admissions

- History of three previous overdoses following breaking up with various boyfriends

- Presents with six episodes of 'fits' in the preceeding month – during each fit she says she experiences loss of consciousness, but no incontinence of urine

- Also presents with suicidal ideas because she has recently separated from her husband

- What is the differential diagnosis and management of this patient?

Answer 12

(a) *Differential diagnosis –*

–   Hysterical personality disorder – most likely diagnosis

–   Need to consider epilepsy

(b) *Management –*

–   Assess suicidal intent – if not thought to be a suicidal risk, discharge from hospital as soon as possible

–   Ongoing supportive psychotherapy (either individual or group) may help the patient to recognize her problems and deal with them more effectively

–   Psychotropic medication may be indicated subsequently if the patient fails to respond to psychological treatment

Question 13

- 30-year-old lady

- Referred from Casualty for a psychiatric opinion

- No previous psychiatric admissions

- Presents with a sudden onset within the last twenty-four hours of global amnesia, paralysis of both arms and abdominal pain, the patient appearing somewhat indifferent towards her symptoms which appear to have been provoked by stressful events

- What is the differential diagnosis and management of this patient?

Answer 13

(a) *Differential diagnosis*

- Hysteria – most likely diagnosis

- Need to consider organic disorder, histrionic personality disorder and malingering

(b) *Management* –

- Admit to hospital for further assessment

- Need to exclude any underlying organic disorder

- Treatment by reassurance and suggestion is usually appropriate, together with immediate efforts to resolve any stressful circumstances that provoked the reaction

- If patient fails to respond to reassurance and suggestion, consider abreacting the patient with an intravenous injection of small amounts of sodium amytal – in the resulting state, the patient is encouraged to relive the stressful events that provoked the hysteria and to express the accompanying emotions.

- The patient may need to be followed up in the Outpatients' Department with dynamic psychotherapy

Question 14

-   55-year-old man

-   Referred by his GP to the Outpatients' Department

-   History of eight previous psychiatric admissions for schizophrenia
    – with the most recent admission about five years ago

-   Presents with a one-month history of the solitary encapsulated
    belief that he is a producing a foul smell from his anus which is
    distressing to other people who come into contact with him

-   What is the differential diagnosis and management of this patient?

Answer 14

(a) *Differential diagnosis –*

– Monosymptomatic delusional psychosis – most likely diagnosis

– Need to consider a relapse of chronic schizophrenia and organic disorder

(b) *Management –*

– Admit to hospital for further assessment

– The patient should be fully investigated physically to ensure that there is no organic basis for the patient's complaint

– The patient should be given a trial of the drug pimozide, which it is claimed in the literature has success in specifically targeting monosymptomatic hypochondriacal delusions

– The patient should be referred to a clinical psychologist for behaviour therapy, which is also claimed to help this condition

– Follow up in the Outpatients' Department

Question 15

- 44-year-old lady

- Referred by her GP to the Outpatients' Department

- No previous psychiatric admissions

- Presents with a four-month history of feeling depressed, panic attacks several times a day accompanied by the feeling that she is going to die, the inability to experience pleasure and loss of energy

- What is the differential diagnosis and management of this patient?

Answer 15

(a) *Differential diagnosis –*

–   Depressive disorder with secondary panic symptoms – most likely diagnosis

–   Need to consider primary panic disorder

(b) *Management –*

–   Treat patient as an outpatient with an antidepressant drug which specifically targets panic symptoms, e.g. fluvoxamine (a 5-HT reuptake inhibitor)

–   If patient fails to respond to antidepressant medication, consider a course of ECT (which should be administered as an inpatient)

–   Follow up in the Outpatients' Department

Question 16

- 25-year-old man

- Referred from the Casualty Department for a psychiatric opinion

- Hisotry of two previous psychiatric admissions for schizophrenia

- Presents with a history of hearing voices commenting on his actions in the third person, hearing voices speaking to him making derisive comments, experiencing that free will is removed and that his behaviour is controlled by some external force, feeling depressed and suicidal ideation

- What is the differential diagnosis and management of this patient?

Answer 16

(a) *Differential diagnosis* –

–   Schizophrenia – most likely diagnosis

–   Need to consider schizoaffective disorder

(b) *Management* –

–   Admit to hospital

–   Immediate management:

   (i)   Administer chlorpromazine (oral or parenteral) in large doses

   (ii)   If no improvement after about two weeks – consider a course of ECT in view of the depressive component to this presentation

   (iii) Patient needs to be carefully observed by nursing staff until his obvious distress and suicidal ideation have departed

–   Long-term management:

   (i)   Patient should be established on a depot injection (e.g. depixol)

   (ii)   On discharge, patient should be followed up by a Community Psychiatric Nurse, who should continue these injections and provide social support for the patient and family

Question 17

–   16-year-old girl

–   Referred by her GP to the Outpatients' Department

–   No previous psychiatric admissions

–   Presents with a two-month history of weight loss, a fear of being fat, the belief that she is too fat even when severely underweight, bulimia and the relentless pursuit of a low body weight

–   What is the differential diagnosis and management of this patient?

Answer 17

(a) *Differential diagnosis* –

– Anorexia nervosa – most likely diagnosis

– Need to consider organic disorder, phobic anxiety neurosis, obsessive compulsive disorder, depressive disorder and schizophrenia

(b) *Management* –

– Admit to hosptital for further assessment

– Need to exclude any underlying organic disorder

– Need to exclude any underlying functional psychiatric illness

– An essential first priority is the maintenance of an adequate weight – a strict regime of refeeding is carried out using a carefully controlled calorie intake

– Chlorpromazine and tricyclic antidepressants may be used to promote weight gain

– Supportive psychotherapy may be used to try to improve the patient's personal relationships and increase her sense of personal effectiveness

– The patient may need to be followed up in the Outpatients' Department with cognitive behaviour therapy, aimed at changing the patient's attitude towards eating, and reappraisal of her self-image and life circumstances

Question 18

–   42-year-old man

–   Taken to Casualty on Section 136 of the MHA 1983 by the police – following an episode of violent behaviour when he threw his television set through the window and physically assaulted his wife

–   History of two previous psychiatric admissions over the last ten years – following overdosing on benzodiazepines

–   History of epilepsy since childhood, currently stabilized on anticonvulsant medication

–   Presents to Casualty with a history of feeling that people may be against him, hearing muffled voices speaking inside his head, a withdrawn appearance, and a low threshold for frustration

–   What is the differential diagnosis and management of this patient?

Answer 18

(a) *Differential diagnosis* –

– Antisocial personality disorder – most likely diagnosis

– Need to consider epilepsy

(b) *Management* –

– Admit to hospital for further assessment and to prevent further episodes of violent behaviour which might occur should he return home

– Reassess his epilepsy by measuring the serum level of his anticonvulsant medication and making any necessary changes to the drug dosage – the latter might include referral to the Neurology Outpatients' Department for advice

– If the violent behaviour continues in hospital, the patient may need to be nursed either in a seclusion room or on a psychiatric intensive therapy unit (ITU), with the administration of parenteral neuroleptics (e.g. dropiderol) and/or benzodiazepines (e.g. lorazepam)

– It may be necessary to seek the advice of a forensic psychiatrist with respect to the management of such violent behaviour in the general psychiatric hospital setting and whether the patient may need transfer to a secure unit

Question 19

- 25-year-old lady

- Referred by her GP to the Outpatients' Department

- No previous psychiatric admissions

- History of premorbidly being inclined to be moody and depressed

- Presents with a two-month history of becoming increasingly preoccupied with the 'large' size of her nose, feeling tense and anxious, and requesting plastic surgery to correct this physical deformity

- Also presents with a two-week history of feeling depressed with self-pity

- What is the differential diagnosis and management of this patient?

Answer 19

(a) *Differential diagnosis –*

- Dysmorphophobia in the context of a vulnerable personality – most likely diagnosis

- Need to consider depressive disorder, schizophrenia and personality disorder

(b) *Management –*

- Reassure the patient that her physical appearance is within normal limits

- See patient for weekly supportive psychotherapy in the Outpatients' Department

- Consider a therapeutic trial of antidepressant medication if patient doesn't improve, on the assumption that she might have an underlying depressive disorder

- If patient is unresponsive to antidepressants, consider admission to hospital for further assessment and management including:

  (i) A course of ECT

  (ii) A therapeutic trial of neuroleptic medication

  (iii) More intensive psychotherapy

Question 20

- 53-year-old man

- Referred by a consultant cardiologist to the Psychiatric Outpatients' Department

- No previous psychiatric admissions

- History of three myocardial infarctions over the last eleven years, with a successful coronary artery bypass operation shortly after his third infarction two years ago

- Presents with a four-month history of feeling depressed, feeling isolated and worry about chest pain

- What is the differential diagnosis and management of this patient?

Answer 20

(a) *Differential diagnosis –*

– Normal reaction to on-going stress – most likely diagnosis

– Need to consider a reactive depression in relation to physical illness

(b) *Management –*

– Admit to the psychiatric day hospital – for further assessment and social support

– If no improvement – start on an antidepressant drug with no clinically significant cardiovascular side-effects (e.g. a 5-HT reuptake inhibitor such as fluvoxamine)

Question 21

- 40-year-old man

- Referred from Casualty for a psychiatric opinion

- History of two previous admissions for detoxification from barbiturates

- Presents to Casualty with a short history of clouding of consciousness, disorientation, major seizures, anxiety, restlessness, pyrexia and tremulousness

- What is the differential diagnosis and management of this patient?

Answer 21

(a) *Differential diagnosis –*

- Withdrawal effects from barbiturates – most likely diagnosis

- Need to consider withdrawal effects from alcohol and withdrawal effects from benozodiazepines

(b) *Management –*

- Admit to hospital

- Exclude alcohol dependence and benzodiazepine dependence

- Detoxify from barbiturates:

    (i) Dosage reduction of barbiturate

    (ii) Cover withdrawal symptoms with a benzodiazepine

    (iii) Use anticonvulsants if necessary

- Aim to rehabilitate the patient by way of:

    (i) Providing him with the interest and support of a caring person

    (ii) Attending to accommodation and work issues

- The patient may need to be followed up with group psychotherapy

Question 22

- 27-year-old lady

- Referred by her GP to the Outpatients' Department

- History of two previous psychiatric admissions for schizophrenia treated with fluspirilene injections

- Presents with a one-month history of prolonged hand washing rituals and compulsive checking rituals following non-compliance with her depot medication for three months

- What is the differential diagnosis and management of this patient?

Answer 22

(a) *Differential diagnosis –*

– Schizophrenic relapse heralded in by obsessive compulsive symptoms – most likely diagnosis

– Need to consider primary OCD (obsessive compulsive disorder)

(b) *Management –*

– Admit to hospital

– Re-establish back on fluspirilene depot medication administered weekly

– Follow up in the Outpatients' Department

Question 23

- 68-year-old lady

- Referred by her GP for an urgent domiciliary visit

- History of one previous psychiatric admission for senile dementia

- Presents with a history of believing that people are against her, feeling depressed, poor concentration, impairment of short-term memory, and temporal and spatial disorientation

- Her husband is unable to cope with her

- What is the differential diagnosis and management of this patient?

Answer 23

(a) *Differential diagnosis –*

- Organic psychosis (i.e. senile dementia with an associated paranoid state) – most likely diagnosis

- Need to consider paraphrenia, depressive disorder and paranoid personality disorder

(b) *Management –*

- Admit to hospital, either informally or under the powers of the Mental Health Act 1983

- Immediate management – thioridazine in moderate doses to reduce the intensity of the persecutory delusions

- Long-term management – social support for husband to help him cope in the form of:

    (i)   Home visits by a Community Psychiatric Nurse

    (ii) Patient attendance at a psychogeriatric day hospital

    (iii) Meals On Wheels

    (iv) Home Help

    (v)   Patient attendance at the Outpatients' Department

    (vi) Small maintenance dose of thioridazine to prevent re-emergence of persecutory delusions

- Ultimately, the patient may require long-term hospitalization

Question 24

- 40-year-old man

- Referred from Casualty for a psychiatric opinion

- History of three previous psychiatric admissions, diagnosed at different times as suffering from alcohol dependence, depressive disorder and paranoid state

- Presents to Casualty with a two-month history of believing his wife has been unfaithful to him and believing his children are plotting against him, and a one-week history of alcohol abuse and feeling depressed

- What is the differential diagnosis and management of this patient?

Answer 24

(a) *Differential diagnosis* –

– Simple paranoid state – most likely diagnosis

– Need to consider alcohol dependence and depressive disorder

(b) *Management* –

– Admit to hospital for further assessment – including an assessment of the degree of the patient's problem with alcohol and the degree of depression

– Detoxify from alcohol

– If clinically depressed, treat with antidepressant medication or ECT

– Treat the underlying paranoid state with antipsychotic medication – patient should be offered this in oral form (e.g. chlorpromazine tablets) but may be reluctant to take it, believing that it might harm him; it may then be necessary to prescribe depot neuroleptic medication (e.g. fluphenazine decanoate injections)

– The psychiatrist should show compassionate interest in the patient's beliefs, but without condemning them or colluding in them

– Follow up in the Psychiatric Outpatients' Department

Question 25

- 25-year-old man

- Taken to Casualty on Section 136 of the MHA 1983 by the police – found indiscriminately attacking people in the street

- No previous psychiatric admissions

- Presents to Casualty in an agitated manner, verbally abusive, screaming and shouting, and threatening to punch the nursing staff

- What is the differential diagnosis and management of this patient?

Answer 25

(a) *Differential diagnosis –*

- That of acutely disturbed behaviour – head injury, metabolic disturbance, prescribed drugs, alcohol or drug dependence, schizophrenia, hypomania and personality disorder

(b) *Management –*

- Admit to hospital for further assessment

- Provide a calm, reassuring and consistent environment in which provocation is avoided

- A special ward area with an adequate number of experienced staff is much better than the use of heavy medication

- If this fails to bring the acutely disturbed behaviour under immediate control, physical restraint and medication may be needed:

    (i) Up to 30 mg of haloperidol may be given intramuscularly in a single dose for emergency control

    (ii) The patient may be given, in addition, an intravenous injection of 4 mg of lorazepam

- Once the acutely disturbed behaviour is under immmediate control, the underlying cause can then be determined

Question 26

- 45-year-old lady

- Referred from Casualty for a psychiatric opinion

- No previous psychiatric admissions

- Presents to Casualty with gross cognitive impairment in clear consciousness, global amnesia, fatuous behaviour, loss of initiative, loss of ethical standards, nominal aphasia and generalized hyperalgesia

- What is the differential diagnosis and management of this patient?

Answer 26

(a) *Differential diagnosis* –

– Pre-senile dementia due to Pick's disease – most likely diagnosis

– Need to consider possible causes of pre-senile dementia where treatment can have a marked benefit (e.g. normal pressure hydrocephalus, hypocalcaemia, hypothyroidism, cerebral tumour, subdural haematoma or alcohol intoxication)

(b) *Management* –

– Admit patient to hospital for further assessment – a psychogeriatric ward may well be the most appropriate setting to assess this patient

– The patient should be fully investigated physically to ensure that no underlying treatable cause of pre-senile dementia is missed

– Such physical assessment should include a full physical examination, skull X-ray, EEG, CT scan of the brain, urea and electrolytes tests, liver function tests and thyroid function tests

– If no treatable cause can be detected, the patient should receive psychometric testing administered by a clinical psychologist, to assess the degree of the patient's confusion

– If ongoing hospitalization is thought to be inevitable in this patient, then she should be placed on a ward where staff engage in reality orientation, to maximize her potential

Question 27

-   25-year-old lady

-   Referred from Casualty for a psychiatric opinion

-   History of two previous psychiatric admissions for schizophrenia in the last four years

-   History of recently abusing LSD, cannabis and amphetamines

-   Presents with a one-month history of hearing voices commenting on her actions and experiencing that her thoughts are being taken out of her mind by some external force

-   What is the differential diagnosis and management of this patient?

Answer 27

(a) *Differential diagnosis –*

– Schizophrenic relapse precipitated by drug abuse – most likely diagnosis

– Need to consider a drug-induced psychosis

(b) *Management –*

– Admit to hospital for further assessment

– Screen urine to confirm illicit drug abuse

– Prescribe depot neuroleptic medication for the patient

– Counsel patient about the dangers of illicit drug abuse

– After discharge, a Community Psychiatric Nurse can continue to:

   (i)   Administer depot injections

   (ii) Monitor the mental state of the patient

   (iii) Liaise with the hospital

Question 28

- 47-year-old lady

- Referred by her GP for a domicillary visit

- No previous psychiatric admissions

- Presents with a three-month history of feeling depressed, compulsive washing of the hands and checking rituals, loss of appetite, loss of weight, initial and middle insomnia and poor concentration

- What is the differential diagnosis and management of this patient?

Answer 28

(a) *Differential diagnosis –*

– Depressive disorder with secondary obsessive compulsive symptoms – most likely diagnosis

– Need to consider primary OCD (obsessive compulsive disorder)

(b) *Management –*

– Treat patient as an outpatient with an antidepressant drug which specifically targets obsessional symptoms, e.g. fluvoxamine (a 5-HT reuptake inhibitor)

– If patient fails to respond to antidepressant medication, consider a course of ECT (which should be administered as an inpatient)

– Follow up in the Outpatients' Department

Question 29

- 40-year-old lady

- Referred by her GP to the Outpatients' Department

- History of two previous psychiatric admissions for depressive disorder

- Presents with a two-month history of a relapse of depressive disorder unresponsive to clomipramine 250 mg nocte taken for six weeks

- What is the management of this patient?

Answer 29

Management –

- Admit to hospital for further assessment

- Exclude any underlying organic disorder

- Attend to any supposed psychosocial factors in the aetiology of the illness

- Add in lithium carbonate (250 mg bd) to the clomipramine

- If patient fails to respond to lithium and clomipramine, consider a course of ECT

- If patient fails to respond to ECT, consider adding in sodium valproate (200 mg bd) to lithium and clomipramine

- Follow up in the Outpatients' Department and continue the antidepressant medication for twelve months post-clinical recovery

Question 30

- 65-year-old man

- Referred by his GP to the Outpatients' Department

- No previous psychiatric admissions

- History of recent positive serology for syphilis treated with a course of penicillin injections at the STD clinic

- Presents with a four-month history of confusion, depression, loss of appetite, early morning wakening, loss of interest in life and psychomotor retardation following his retirement

- What is the differential diagnosis and management of this patient?

Answer 30

(a) *Differential diagnosis –*

– Depressive disorder – most likely diagnosis

– Need to consider GPI (general paralysis of the insane)

(b) *Management –*

– Admit to hospital for further assessment

– Re-refer to STD clinic

– Treat depressive disorder with an alerting antidepressant drug in view of the psychomotor retardation (e.g. lofepramine or fluoxetine)

– If patient fails to respond to antidepressant medication, consider a course of ECT

– Ensure patient has adequate social support networks outside hospital when discharged

Question 31

- 40-year-old man

- Taken to Casualty on Section 136 of the MHA 1983 by the police – following a suicide attempt when he tried to kill himself by jumping in front of a car

- History of three previous psychiatric admissions over the last eight years following wrist slashing

- History of alcohol dependence, drug dependence on lorazepam and a forensic history for shoplifting and housebreaking

- Presents to Casualty with a strong smell of alcohol, marked agitation, verbal abuse directed towards the nursing staff and feelings of depression

- Currently homeless and unemployed

- What is the differential diagnosis and management of this patient?

Answer 31

(a) *Differential diagnosis –*

–   Antisocial personality disorder with associated alcohol/drug dependence – most likely diagnosis

–   Need to consider alcohol/drug dependence as the primary diagnosis

(b) *Management –*

–   Admit to hospital for further assessment – including assessment of suicidal risk and assessment of the degree of his alcohol/drug dependence

–   Detoxify from alcohol

–   Substitute diazepam (long-acting) for lorazepam (short-acting) and then gradually decrease and stop the former

–   Assess mood once detoxified from alcohol and benzodiazepines – if clinically depressed, treat with an antidepressant drug or a course of ECT as appropriate

–   Discharge to an after-care hostel specialising in patients treated for alcohol dependence

–   Refer him to the DRO (Disablement Resettlement Officer) to help him find employment

–   Follow up in the Psychiatric Outpatients' Department to encourage and support him not to revert back to substance abuse

Question 32

–   45-year-old man

–   Taken to Casualty on Section 136 of the MHA 1983 by the police – having attacked two of his neighbours

–   No previous psychiatric admissions

–   History of being hypersensitive all his life and being unable to accept even mild criticism

–   Presents with a sudden onset of believing that his neighbours are talking about him and criticising him and hearing the muffled voices of his two neighbours talking to each other about him, having recently separated from his wife

–   What is the differential diagnosis and management of this patient?

Answer 32

(a) *Differential diagnosis* –

–   Paranoid personality disorder – most likely diagnosis

–   Need to consider schizophrenia

(b) *Management* –

–   Admit to hospital for further assessment – including an assessment of what danger from violence the patient presents to others

–   Immediate management – oral anxiolytic drugs or neuroleptic medication may be given for short periods, as this is a time of unusual stress for the patient

–   Long-term management – depot neuroleptic medication may be helpful in preventing relapse of a paranoid personality disorder

–   Supervision and support may be benenficial – can be given by a Community Psychiatric Nurse or social worker

–   Future admissions to hospital should be avoided whenever possible, but may be necessary for short periods of crisis

Question 33

– 30-year-old man

– Referred by his GP to the Outpatients' Department

– History of two previous psychiatric admissions for schizophrenia

– Presents with a two-month history of a relapse of schizophrenia with positive symptoms, unresponsive to chlorpromazine 100 mg tds taken for six weeks

– What is the management of this patient?

Answer 33

Management –

– Admit to hospital for further assessment

– Exclude any underlying organic disorder

– Attend to any supposed psychosocial factors in the aetiology of the illness

– Increase the oral dosage of chlorpromazine up to 250 mg qds

– If the patient fails to respond to this dosage of chlorpromazine, consider adding in an antipsychotic depot injection (e.g. flupenthixol decanoate)

– If patient fails to respond to chlorpromazine and depot, consider stopping the depot and adding in clozepine tablets

– Follow up in the Outpatients' Department, ensuring that the patient has regular blood tests to detect any possible agranulocytosis (life-threatening side-effect of clozepine)

Question 34

–   25-year-old lady

–   Referred by her GP to the Outpatients' Department

–   History of two previous psychiatric admissions for depressive disorder

–   Presents with feeling depressed, irritable, agitated and aggressive – the symptoms occurring periodically in relation to the onset of menstruation

–   What is the differential diagnosis and management of this patient?

Answer 34

(a) *Differential diagnosis* –

- PMS (premenstrual syndrome) – most likely diagnosis

- Need to consider depressive disorder

(b) *Management* –

- Refer for hormonal assay – to detect any related hormonal imbalance

- Therapeutic trial of various hormonal tablets (e.g. the oral contraceptive pill)

- Therapeutic trial of an antidepressant tablet

- Pyridoxine (vitamin B$_6$) may also be useful

- Supportive psychotherapy

Question 35

- 50-year-old lady

- Referred from Casualty for a psychiatric opinion

- No previous psychiatric admissions

- Presents to Casualty with palpitations, fearful anticipation, irritability, a feeling of restlessness, agitation, tachycardia and a coarse tremor of the hands

- What is the differential diagnosis and management of this patient?

Answer 35

(a) *Differential diagnosis –*

–   Anxiety neurosis – most likely diagnosis

–   Need to consider depressive disorder, schizophrenia and organic disorders in which anxiety symptoms occur (e.g. alcohol and drug abuse, thyrotoxicosis, phaeochromocytoma and hypoglycaemia

(b) *Management –*

–   Admit to hospital for further assessment

–   Exclude an organic disorder by carrying out a full physical assessment

–   Exclude an ongoing anxiety provoking factor in the patient's home or family life (i.e. current situational stresses) by referring the patient to a social worker for a full psychosocial assessment

–   Admission to hospital and reassurance may in themselves be beneficial to the patient without physical treatment being necessary

–   If hospitalization and reassurance do not prove beneficial, physical treatment should be considered:

    (i)   Benzodiazepines (e.g. diazepam) provide symptomatic relief of anxiety in the short-term, but should not be prescribed for more than a few weeks

    (ii) If medication has to be prolonged for more than a few weeks, it is appropriate to prescribe a tricyclic antidepressant which is effective due to its anxiolytic properties (e.g. prothiaden)

–   Follow up at the Outpatients' Department

Question 36

- 82-year-old lady

- Referred by her GP to the Outpatients' Department

- No previous psychiatric admissions

- History of angina and hypertension

- Presents with a one-month history of sudden onset of confusion, temporal and spatial disorientation, impairment of short-term memory, depression and agitation

- What is the differential diagnosis and management of this patient?

Answer 36

(a) *Differential diagnosis –*

- Multi-infarct dementia – most likely diagnosis

- Need to consider SDAT (senile dementia of the Alzheimer's type), cardiac failure and depressive disorder

(b) *Management –*

- Admit to psychogeriatric day hospital for attendance – two to three days per week

- Arrange for Community Psychiatric Nurse to visit patient at home for support

- Arrange for Home Help

- Essential to provide encouragement and support for her caring relatives

- Therapeutic trial of a non-cardiotoxic antidepressant (e.g. fluvoxamine) may prove useful

Question 37

–   35-year-old lady

–   Referred by her GP to the Outpatients' Department

–   History of two previous psychiatric admissions for hypomania

–   Presents with a two-month history of a relapse of hypomania unresponsive to haloperidol 5 mg qds taken for six weeks

–   What is the management of this patient?

Answer 37

Management –

- Admit to hospital for further assessment

- Exclude any underlying organic disorder

- Attend to any psychosocial factors that may be aetiological in the illness

- Increase the oral dosage of haloperidol up to 50 mg qds

- If patient fails to respond to this dosage of haloperidol, consider adding in lithium carbonate (but do not exceed 20 mg qds of haloperidol in combination with lithium, because of the risk of neuroleptic malignant syndrome)

- If patient fails to respond to lithium and haloperidol, consider stopping the lithium and adding in carbamazepine

- If patient fails to respond to carbamazepine and haloperidol, the following strategies may be considered:

  (i) Substituting droperidol for haloperidol

  (ii) Substituting sodium valproate for carbamazepine

  (iii) Adding in an antipsychotic depot injection (NB – depot medication certainly protects against hypomanic relapse, but whether it also protects aginast a subsequent depressive relapse of a bipolar affective disorder is not entirely clear)

  (iv) A course of ECT

- Follow up patient in the Outpatients' Department

Question 38

–   25-year-old lady

–   Referred from Casualty for a psychiatric opinion

–   History of two previous psychiatric admissions for depressive
    disorder and acute alcohol withdrawal respectively

–   Presents with a two-month history of feeling depressed, drinking
    up to half a bottle of spirits a day, loss of appetite and loss of
    weight, with a 'fit' at home just before being taken to Casualty

–   What is the differential diagnosis and management of this patient?

Answer 38

(a) *Differential diagnosis* –

–   Depressive disorder with associated alcohol dependence – most likely diagnosis

–   Need to consider alcohol dependence as the primary diagnosis

(b) *Management* –

–   Admit to hospital for further assessment – including an assessment of the degree of alcohol dependence

–   Detoxify from alcohol

–   Treat depressive disorder with physical treatment as appropriate (antidepressant medication or ECT)

–   Refer patient to Alcoholics Anonymous

–   Follow up in the Psychiatric Outpatients' Department

Question 39

- 75-year-old lady

- Referred by her GP to the Outpatients' Department

- No previous psychiatric admissions

- History of right hip replacement five years ago for osteoarthritis

- Presents with a six-month history of back pain, paraesthesia in her right leg, poor hearing, headache, visual disturbance, constipation, feeling depressed and middle insomnia

- What is the differential diagnosis and management of this patient?

Answer 39

(a) *Differential diagnosis* –

– Depressive disorder with secondary hypochondriasis – most likely diagnosis

– Need to consider organic disorder and primary hypochondriasis

(b) *Management* –

– Admit to psychogeriatric day hospital – for further assessment and to provide a social outlet for the patient

– A full physical examination together with appropriate physical investigations should be carried out to exclude an underlying organic disorder and to reassure the patient that her problems are being attended to thoroughly

– Treat patient with an antidepressant drug with minimal physical side-effects (e.g. a 5-HT reuptake inhibitor or a tetracyclic antidepressant)

– If patient fails to respond to antidepressant medication, consider a course of ECT

– Seek the help of the patient's family in managing her

– The patient should continue on antidepressant medication for six months post-clinical recovery for prophylaxis

Question 40

- 30-year-old lady

- Referred by her GP to the Outpatients' Department

- History of two previous psychiatric admissions for depressive disorder which responded to Prothiaden

- Presents with panic attacks associated with feelings of unreality about herself and her environment, feeling depressed, loss of appetite, loss of weight and diffuse anxiety

- What is the differential diagnosis and management of this patient?

Answer 40

(a) *Differential diagnosis* –

–   Phobic anxiety depersonalization syndrome – most likely diagnosis

–   Need to consider depressive disorder

(b) *Management* –

–   Treat patient as an outpatient with Prothiaden (which she
    previously responded to)

–   If she failed to respond to this drug, it would be worthwhile
    treating her with a non-alerting 5-HT reuptake inhibitor (e.g.
    fluvoxamine)

–   She would need to attend the Outpatients' Department at periodic
    intervals for several months